Ashley Fitzgerald

HEALTH:
MICRO HABITS
for
MACRO WELL BEING

New health rules to get boundless energy and achieve body and mind wellness.

Exercise. Yoga. Meditation. Qi Gong. Self and partner massage. Health food

Published by UNITEXTO

TABLE OF CONTENTS

Introduction:

This age presents new challenges and possibilities for mankind. While we have technology to thank for new opportunities for work and for free time, we have also acquired unhealthy habits, such as spending unprecedented amounts of our lives in a seated position. We lack time, and so turn to fast food options and stay seated from morning to night. On the other hand, we know this isn't healthy. We need solutions that are in line with the demands of our lives and are effective for bringing us well-being and keeping us in that state.

What we can do is incorporate ancient practices such as meditation, Yoga, Qi Gong and simple diet adjustments in to our lives. This takes little time, and is very easy and absolutely do-able for anyone.

For example, five to ten minutes of meditation every morning and evening can serve to eradicate stress. A 30 minute Yoga routine in the morning, afternoon or night can make all the difference in the world between a healthy and fit body, and a sluggish and ailing one. Qi Gong can boost our energy and help us sleep. A healthy diet high in organic fruits and vegetables will help the body to cleanse itself of impurities and to rejuvenate itself. We will lose weight in the process and experience glowing health.

This book will show you how to make small adjustments with minimal effort to affect maximum results using small diet changes and short exercise routines. As an added bonus, you will learn some massage techniques to help your body to detox itself, and also some techniques you can practice with a partner for fun, well-being and relaxation.

This is a health book for fast-paced, modern times. This is a collection of practices that have withstood the test of time and are ready to be implemented by those who really need them!

Chapter 1: A Healthy Attitude (How state of mind affects the body and choices which can harm or help)

Everyone wants to feel good, have a healthy body which looks and feels great. Everyone also wants to have a happy state of mind. The two go hand in hand. If you feel great physically, your chances of mental happiness are higher. If you are happy in mind, your body will also follow. Work on one, the other will follow, work on both, everything will fall into place.

Sometimes it's hard to know where to start. Start with your mind. If you can cultivate happiness from within, you can get motivation for action to change other aspects of your life. Practice deep breathing, and let go. Then imagine yourself doing something good for you. Picture yourself drinking a green smoothie instead of eating a bagel for breakfast. See yourself walking on a forest path, swimming in a lake and smiling with friends. Visualize the change you would like to get in your life.

Mental Pathways

Once you create mental pathways for what you are looking to achieve, you will find it easier to put the actions into practice. You will already be familiar with what you are looking to do and will encounter less mental resistance.

The only tool you need to start this path is an open mind. If you are willing to make small changes to bring on huge benefits, then proceed.

What You Need

Other than an open mind and sufficient motivation, you will find it helpful to invest in a Yoga mat and some comfortable clothes to exercise in. Be prepared to shop for healthy organic foods, which do not have to be expensive, and to put in at least 30 minutes each day total for exercise and meditation. More is better, but 30 minutes is the absolute minimum to see results using meditation and exercise.

We wish you much luck and success on your journey to make your life easier and happier!

Chapter 2: On Track to Better Health with Exercise

Working out isn't just about burning calories and losing weight to look good (though this is certainly an important factor!). Exercise helps the joints, prevents arthritis, increases the flow of spinal fluid, increases the amount of oxygen available to the lungs and to the cells of the body, helps the memory, speeds thought processes and releases endorphins which increase feelings of well-being. Exercise can make the difference between living a miserable life, and living a happy and vital one.

Where and How to Get Moving

If you've never had a gym membership or played a sport of any kind, you can still get your body moving easily. A great way to start is just by taking short walks. Instead of driving to the store, walk. Walk to your friends' houses. Take a nature walk in a park or in the woods. Hiking is especially good for you since trees produce oxygen and the unlevel paths cause different parts of the leg muscles to be activated and used than just walking down the street.

Another good way to get started is by doing toe raises while brushing your teeth or while standing up on the subway or on a bus. Just raise yourself up onto your toes and then lower yourself again. Repeat this several times. This increases the circulation in your legs and strengthens the calf muscles.

Getting Inspired for Exercise

Find a sport you really love, and then do it passionately. If you like the company of others, join a team and play softball, baseball or soccer(football), volleyball or tennis. You can just hit a tennis ball back and forth between a friend while chatting.

If you need time alone, then start doing jogging or swimming at an indoor pool. You can swim laps while concentrating simply on your breath. You will clear your mind, exercise you body and feel refreshed and rejuvenated afterwards.

If you've always wanted to try rock climbing, go to a climbing hall where you can find everything you need to start. The controlled environment makes it easy to overcome fears and get started. Then you can progress to climbing outdoors.

Buy a bike or pull out your bike and go for a trip in the countryside. Take a healthy lunch and go for a picnic. Go biking alone or with your family or some friends. Go to the beach and go swimming and take walks in the sand. Walking on sand exercises the whole leg and results in good-looking, strong and toned legs.

Take a Yoga class or a pilates class. Try Zumba or another type of dancing. Go in-line skating, ice skating or give cross country skiing a try. Go boating or diving if you love the water. Try weight lifting if you want to build up muscle mass.

There are so many ways to exercise your body, you are sure to find something that appeals to you!

Chapter 3: How Yoga Makes You Feel Better

Yoga has become an increasingly popular past time. We can't call it a sport, since it is so much more than that. It is thousands of years old, but has only been practiced in the west for a few decades. It owes its popularity to its effectiveness in toning and trimming the body, bringing relaxation and happiness to practitioners. Some say it opens the doors to a new spiritual worldview. Others start a more active lifestyle after beginning Yoga. Whatever effects it has on individuals, everyone agrees that these are positive.

The Power of the Breath
One of the ways Yoga works is in connecting the breath with movements. Whatever motion you make, you connect it with either an inhalation or an exhalation. This way the cells of the body have enough oxygen available. This energizes the body and relaxes the mind. Let's take a look at a few simple Yoga exercises to get started with. You can do them right at home. Comfortable, not too loose and not too tight clothing is recommended as is a Yoga mat which can be purchased online or at most department stores or specialty shops.

A Simple Yoga Pose to Start With

1. Stand up straight.
2. Inhale and lift your shoulders, bring them back and feel your shoulder blades moving down.
3. Relax and look forward and exhale.
4. Now inhale, and bring your arms up over your head.
5. Exhale and bring your arms down.
6. Repeat this several times and end with the hands in prayer pose.

Downward Facing Dog: An Exercise to Do Every Single Day

If you do no other Yoga today, do this pose. It wakes up and strengthens the arm and leg muscles, helps to relax the mind, eases tension in the shoulders, aids in circulation and opens up the hips and gives a nice stretch to the hamstrings. It is an amazing way to warm up before going jogging, or practicing any other sport.

1. Put your hands on the floor shoulder width apart.
2. Inhale and step back and lift your hips, bending your knees.
3. Slowly lower your heels toward the floor while exhaling.

4. The hands are pushing against the mat, and spread your fingers to activate the muscles in your hands.
5. Lift and spread your toes to activate more muscles in the legs. You are in an inverted V shape.
6. Inhale and exhale at least five times in this position, or stay here until you feel great. You can walk out your feet raising the heels and lowering them, sway from side to side, shake your head yes and no to release tension from the neck. This is a crucial pose to any Yoga practice.

Some Other Yoga Poses to Stretch and Strengthen the Body

Plank Pose

1. With your hands shoulder's width apart on the mat, step your feet back into a raised push up position while inhaling.
2. Exhale and tighten your abdominal muscles. Inhale and exhale and repeat, maintaining this position. Spread your toes and feel the lift behind your knees.

Low lunge

1. From a downward facing dog pose, raise your right leg while inhaling.
2. Keep your hips squared and bring the right foot in toward your chest.
3. Now bring it in between your hands and straighten the left leg.
4. Inhale, exhale and repeat on the other side. This is a wonderful way to stretch out your hips.

Yoga makes you feel better because it focuses on the breath. The breath is a source of energy for the body and is also relaxing. Have you ever wondered why you should count to ten and breathe when you are angry? The breath helps to relax the mind and active other parts of the brain. An easy and deep breath will keep you feeling great. Adding the movements to the breath keeps the body limber and in good shape.

Chapter 4: Meditation Grows Brain Cells and Brings Relaxation

Meditation isn't just a "New Age" spiritual practice. Science has found that it really does bring a whole slew of benefits to the mind and body. Among these findings is the confirmation the meditation relieves stress and aids in memory recall. Some people claim that meditation aids in the creation of gray mass in the brain and that it helps to restore brain cells. At the very least, it doesn't damage them! Indeed, a relaxed body and mind allow the body to optimally perform all of the processes it needs to maintain and protect health and well-being.

If you've never tried to meditate, you can start now, at this present moment. It is very easy, and doesn't have to take long. (As you become used to it, you can lengthen meditation sessions). You can also try guided meditations to start with. There are many good ones for specific purposes on YouTube. For example, you can do a guided meditation for relaxation, for healing, and for other specific goals. The point here is to influence the subconscious into enacting positive change. Classic meditation however, consists of slowing or stopping the thoughts.

How to Meditate

1. To get started, find a comfortable place and a comfortable position to sit down or lie down. If you can't get comfortable sitting down, trying lying down. Be careful with lying down, however, since it's easy to fall asleep this way. You want to stay alert and aware while meditating. Your thoughts will slow down to the phase of brain activity you enter right before falling asleep, but you do NOT want to fall asleep when meditating. (With guided meditations, it's acceptable to fall asleep.)

2. Once you've made yourself comfortable, begin breathing deeply. Take full inhales and exhale all of the air out of your lungs.

3. Repeat this and become lost in the rhythm of your breathing. You have nowhere to go, nothing to do. You simply are, and this is perfect. Feel the breath, rising and falling, rising and falling like the tide of the ocean. It is hypnotic and calming, yet you remain fully aware of it. Stay this way for five minutes minimum, and longer if it feels right.

Another way to bring one's self into a meditative state is the following method.

1. Start out by lying down or sitting down in a comfortable position that doesn't cause you to fall asleep.
2. Breathe deeply as in the above method, but this time picture a number 10 in your mind's eye. Inhale, exhale and then picture a number 9. Repeat this process down through all of the remaining numbers, from 8 to 1.
3. Repeat by restarting at 10 if you so desire, to deepen the state. Then simply observe your thoughts coming and going.

Chapter 5: Qi Gong Improves Health, Gives You an Energy Boost and Helps You to Sleep Well

Qi Gong is an ancient practice China which is designed to increase energy in the body. This energy is called Qi, or chi. (In Yoga, life energy is called Prana). The benefits of having more energy are numerous. You feel more capable and stronger when just going about your daily activities. Your immune system becomes much more resistant, so you will find yourself getting colds and other ailments much less often.

Qi Gong is a wonderful and relaxing way to bring more energy into your body. It is gentle and appropriate for all ages, whether you are young or very old, whether you are an athlete or suffer from arthritis or multiple sclerosis, you will find Qi Gong to be helpful in limbering up the body and giving you more energy.

Here are some easy exercises you can try at home.

Feeling Free (Qi Gong Exercise)

1. Sit in a chair with your feet flat on the floor or with your legs crossed on a Yoga mat or a comfortable rug on the floor. Feel grounding through your feet or from the base of your spine.

2. Sit up straight while taking a deep breath. Exhale and relax (but don't slouch). Your neck is relaxed, and your head and entire back feel free.
3. Now inhale and bring your arms out to the sides at shoulder height. Exhale and lower them slowly. Repeat.

Ball of Energy
The concept of the ball of energy will appear repeatedly in Qi Gong exercises

Visualize a ball of energy between your two hands. Hold your hands as if you are really holding a ball, with one hand on top and one below. Roll the ball around, sense it between your hands (but don't "squeeze" the ball or move your hands through it). Really feel the energy.

Lifting the Sky Qi Gong Exercise
The Lifting the Sky exercise is many people's favorite. Some say it has changed their lives for the better!

1. Stand with your feet close together, the mouth open slightly and your toes facing forward. Your hands should be relaxed at the sides. You are standing straight but are completely relaxed.
2. Now have your palms face the ground and point the fingers toward one another. Make sure there

is some space between your fingers. Keep the arms as straight as is comfortable.

3. Now move your arms up over your head while keeping the hands in the same position as number 2. Follow the movement with your nose. Breathe in gently through the nose as you raise the arms.

4. Lower your arms slowly while exhaling out of the mouth. Face forward in a natural way.

5. Repeat.

To experience more of Qi Gong, find some videos to follow along with on YouTube or find an instructor where you live to guide you further. For now, you have some exercises to try right at home that are safe and easy to do.

Chapter 6: Self-Massage and Partner Massage for Lymph Flow and Relaxation

Many people suffer from tense, sore muscles and associated pain. We often think we have to spend a lot of money to get a professional to help. While this is a great way to treat yourself, you can manage aches, pains and tension yourself by doing a self-massage!

How to do a self-massage effectively (step by step):

1. First take a warm bath or a warm shower to loosen up your muscles. Use Epsom salt in the bath if you can, or another type of bath salts.
2. Keep your clothes off if you can. If you cannot have privacy wear light clothing.
3. Use organic massage oil. You can also use olive oil, almond oil, coconut oil or another type of food grade quality oil. Grape seed oil is excellent since it is fragrance free. Coconut oil has anti-viral and anti-fungal properties but smells strong (some people like it and says it smells like "the beach".)
4. Start massaging yourself from the base of the skull down to the shoulders. Massage lightly going in clockwise and then counterclockwise circles. Focus on any areas that feel particularly

tense. Massage the right side of the body with the right hand, the left with the left side.

5. After you've massaged your entire shoulder area, give yourself a hug to stretch out the shoulder blades.

Abdominal Massage to Relieve Menstrual Pain and Improve Digestion

1. Place a hand on the abdomen and massage in a circular motion over the entire area.
2. Apply pressure to different parts of the abdomen using just the tips of the fingers. Hold and then release after a few seconds.

An Effective Back Massage You Can Do On Yourself

Don't have anyone to massage your back? You can still work on your own knots and find relief.

1. Take a ball (preferably a basketball or something on the firmer side.)
2. Stand near a wall and put the ball between your back and the wall.
3. Use the ball to massage your entire back.

Lymph Massage-What is it?

The lymph system transports waste out of the body and is crucial in keeping the system healthy. A highly functional lymph system aids in weight loss. A bogged down lymph system, on the other hand, makes weight loss very difficult. Since it doesn't circulate by itself (as the blood does), it is very beneficial to help it along by massaging areas where lymph is found.

One such area is right at the base of the neck. The cleft where the clavicle begins is a crucial area. When performing a lymph massage, apply only minimal force. Think of the force you need to pull a coin across a table with the tips of the fingers: that's all you need. Put your fingers onto the cleft just at the base of the neck. Pull down slightly with just the lightest touch. Hold for two seconds and release for two seconds. Repeat. This will help to keep the sinuses clear.

Partner Massage
If you are in a relationship, a wonderful thing you can do for your partner and yourself is massage. Some massage oil, time and privacy are all you need. Use circular motions to work out knots on one another in conjunction with your preferred type of massage oil. Take care to not work any areas too hard and respect each other's boundaries. Do not apply pressure to the spine since this could result in injury (if you are a professional you can touch the spinal area, but for beginners it's best to simply avoid this region to ensure

no injury occurs.) Massage is an excellent way to bring lovers closer together and such can serve as therapy for the body, mind and spirit.

Chapter 7: The Role Food Plays on Health (And What to Eat and Drink for Optimal Health)

"You can let your food be your medicine, and your medicine be your food." This is the way of the future. If you eat to support your health you can strengthen your body and avoid debilitating illness.

It has been recommended for too long that a human's diet should consist mainly of carbohydrates. Carbohydrates are broken down as sugars, and an overabundance of sugar is unhealthy for the digestive system, and the entire body. Instead, the diet should concentrate on green vegetables, berries and other low-sugar produce. Healthy fats such as coconut oil, olive oil and organic butter are essential for the body, which may come as a surprise to some. Fat has been given such a bad reputation, but not all fat is bad for you. (Trans fat is still unhealthy, and should be avoided!)

As an example, in the past, farmers were told that fat increases weight. They fed their pigs coconut oil and where astounded when their pigs lost weight, had increased energy and were active and slim! We should take this example, and feed ourselves coconut oil to have increased energy for doing sports and going about our daily lives.

We often don't start to think about what we are putting into our bodies until we feel unwell. Celiac's disease, (the inability to process gluten in the body) leads to many people cutting out bread from their lives and their food. Lactose intolerance leads to the removal of milk products from the diet.

Diabetes forces people to watch their sugar intake. Instead, if you limit your intake of all of these products, you can prevent the onset of these uncomfortable conditions. None of them are essential for the diet. You can substitute goat milk and goat cheese for cow milk and cow milk based cheese. You can switch to organic and gluten free products, and most importantly, limit your sugar intake to a minimal level.

Probiotics for Health

Another reason to cut down on sugar intake is that cancer cells, parasites and fungus all need sugar to survive. All of the above are extremely unhealthy and can lead to the breakdown of the well-being in the body. We want to stop cancer from developing, keep fungus from taking over, and safely get rid of parasites. Eating raw garlic helps to control parasites, and you can find natural products for getting rid of parasites effectively. Ask a health professional if you need consultation on this topic and suspect you may suffer from parasites.

If you've had to take antibiotics for an illness in your life, you may suffer from fungus overgrowth in the body. Why? The healthy bacteria in the body that helps digestion is also killed by antibiotics, not only the invaders that are being targeted. This leads to problems with the normal balance of the body, and the naturally occurring yeast takes over and can damage the gut when it grows out of control. To keep this fungus from making you really ill, you need to limit your sugar intake and take probiotics.

One good way to do this is to stop drinking sugar-laden sodas and replace this with healthy and gut-health promoting Kombucha. Kombucha is a fermented tea that contains healthy bacteria and can be more effective than a probiotic capsule. A great way to make sure you help the regrowth of healthy bacteria is to make your own yoghurt, kefir and Kombucha. You can also make your own sauerkraut. www.iherb.comhas a selection of yoghurt and kefir starters so you can make your own yoghurt and kefir.

You can also buy Kombucha from iherb.com. Probiotic foods are a fundament of maintaining good health and healing after illness. Sometimes it is just unavoidable, and you have to go on antibiotics. The best way you can get your health back afterward is to consume probiotics. (Probiotic means "pro-life", while antibiotic means, "anti-life". Antibiotics kill all of the bacteria in the body, whether good or bad. You need something to reset the balance in the body).

Being Mindful When You Eat
Pay attention to how your food makes you feel while you eat it and after you have eaten. Take small bites, chew slowly and visualize your food healing you and doing your body good. Eating too fast can cause indigestion. Food needs to be properly digested in order to really be able to process vitamins and minerals to be used in the body.

Fat-Soluble Vitamins
In terms of vegetables, it is important to eat them with some form of fat. Many vitamins are only fat-soluble which means the body cannot process them without the presence of some type of oil or fat. This is very simple. When you make a salad, make sure you top it with olive oil or some other type of cold-pressed oil. Add apple cider vinegar to balance the pH in the body. When you eat cooked or steamed vegetables, add butter, ghee or coconut oil. Coconut oil has benefits such as being anti-

microbial and anti-viral. (Though it won't harm your good bacteria!)

Bone Broth Soup for Health

For those who eat meat, try a bone broth soup. The natural collagen and gelatin is excellent for the digestive tract and also for the skin, hair and nails. To make bone broth soup, slow cook bones of beef, chicken or turkey for several hours along with vegetables. Good vegetables for broth include carrots, celeriac, fennel, celery, chives and parsnip. Simply wash, slice and peel them where necessary and add them to the cooking bone broth after a few hours have passed with just the bones cooking. Before serving, remove the bones and add salt and pepper to taste. This is an excellent meal along with a salad and/or gluten free bread.

Healthy, Nourishing Vegetables

Some particularly healthy vegetables include avocado, spinach, kale and asparagus. Avocado is rich in vegetable-based protein (especially important for vegetarians and vegans) and vitamin E. Spinach is also rich in vegetable-based protein, iron, vitamin A, magnesium and potassium. Kale is rich in vitamin K, which is essential for bone health. Asparagus contains vitamin C (essential for the immune system), vitamin K, thiamin, manganese, potassium, selenium, niacin, iron and more.

Asparagus is delicious when steamed and served with butter. Focus on getting a few servings of each of these vegetables every week, or better, every day. Those who eat avocados reportedly are healthier and stronger, with shinier hair and stronger nails. You can add them to a sandwich or a salad, eat them as guacamole in a dip, and more. Add them to smoothies for a creamy consistency.

Asparagus can also be eaten raw, or steamed in a salad accompanied by avocado, tomatoes, baby spinach and kale. Kale can be added to smoothies if you don't like it's texture in a salad. Another tasty way to eat kale is as kale chips. These crispy, air-dried delicacies can be bought at health stores and most conventional supermarkets or made at home if you have a dehydrator. (Look online for recipes).

Meal Ideas
An excellent breakfast consists of homemade yoghurt with low-sugar berries such as strawberries, raspberries and blueberries. You can try making yoghurt with young coconut if you are a vegan. Young Thai coconuts can be purchased at health food stores and Asian food shops (they are much cheaper at Asian

31

food shops.) A healthy lunch consists of vegetable or bone broth soup and a salad or gluten free sandwich.

For dinner, you can eat steamed vegetables and buckwheat noodles, for example. There are many options out there. Try to keep your meals heavy on vegetables and healthy fats, with some source of protein but low on carbohydrates. Drink Kombucha with your meal, and try to include some probiotics food with each meal (whether that is sauerkraut, yoghurt or Kombucha). Drink organic green tea and plenty of water. You will be feeling energetic and healthy in no time.

Chapter 8: General Tips to Bringing More Well-Being into Your Daily Life

The key to feeling better often lies with adjusting your mental world first of all. If you have a positive outlook for life, the rest will usually fall in place. A positive attitude is pre-requisite for changing your health for the better, since motivation is needed to put change into effect. Meditation is a powerful tool toward feeling better. Exercise causes the brain to release endorphins, which are also effective toward creating a positive mood. (Endorphins are also called feel-good hormones).

Changing your diet and eliminating processed foods and reducing sugars can also make you feel better. Each link in the chain is connected. If you improve one area, it will positively affect other areas of your life. If you begin by exercising, you will bring more feel-good hormones into your body. If you meditate, you will have more control over your moods and feelings. If you start out by just changing your thought patterns, you will have more motivation for changing your diet. If you try out new and interesting ways to prepare vegetables and cut out sugar, you will have more energy and more even moods (since you won't experience the crash and burn that sugar causes).

Yoga and Qi Gong will get you breathing more deeply and will thus increase the amount of energy available in your body. All of these elements will help you raise the standards of your life, making your daily world a better place. It may take some effort and small steps to change, but if you get on the path to better health, you will NOT want to go back. (Kombucha is addictive, in a good way!)

If you are feeling down, try cleaning your house and re-organizing things, throwing out what you don't need. The results will have you feeling you have accomplished something. A de-cluttered household will improve your concentration, since a load of clutter is distracting and often irritating.

When feeling too tired for more strenuous exercise, just take a walk. The fresh air is good for the immune system, and movement is good for the joints. You might then be inspired to do some more heavy exercise. In addition, sunshine stimulates the production of Vitamin D in the body (you need sunlight to get vitamin D, and it is more effective to get it through the skin's exposure to the sun than through food). You don't want a sunburn, but daily exposure to the sun is essential for

34

Vitamin D. This also helps the mood and the immune system. (This is reason people often feel depressed in the winter).

If you want to reduce your exposure to chemicals, switch to organic, natural cleaning products or make your own using white vinegar. Switch from plastic bottles to glass. Use organic textiles and eat only organic produce. Do a detox diet whenever possible (a juice feast, or a fast). This will also help to improve your health and your overall mood.

Conclusion

Health is the basis for leading a good, long life. If you feel good because you are healthy, you will have a better foundation for positive, loving relationships and a rewarding job and fun leisure activities. On the other hand, if you feel unwell, it will be hard to have much to contribute to a relationship or on the job. If you are battling illness, you won't have much energy or motivation to do fun things. Create a foundation for good health, and you can look to the future with hope and happiness.